DR. LEO K. MITCHELL

Type 2 Diabetes Natural Prevention Guide

A Step-By-Step Program to Lower Your Risk, Reverse Prediabetes, and Protect Your Health

Contents

About the Author

Dr. Leo K. Mitchell is a renowned expert in the field of preventive medicine and a passionate advocate for promoting health and wellness. With a deep-rooted commitment to helping individuals prevent and manage chronic diseases, Dr. Mitchell has dedicated his career to empowering people to take control of their health and live their best lives.

Throughout his career, Dr. Mitchell has worked closely with patients, guiding them on their journey towards optimal health. He firmly believes in the power of education and empowers his patients with the knowledge and tools they need to make informed decisions about their well-being.

With "Type 2 Diabetes Natural Prevention Guide," Dr. Leo K. Mitchell aims to share his expertise and empower readers to take charge of their health. By offering practical advice, evidence-based strategies, and a compassionate approach, he hopes to inspire individuals to make positive changes and reduce their risk of developing type 2 diabetes.

Introduction

Dear Reader,

Have you ever felt like your health is slipping out of your hands? Like you're on a rollercoaster ride, with your blood sugar levels soaring and plummeting, leaving you feeling exhausted, frustrated, and uncertain about the future? If so, you're not alone.

My name is Dr. Leo K. Mitchell, and I want to share my personal journey with you. A few years ago, I received a life-changing diagnosis: Type 2 Diabetes. It hit me like a ton of bricks, and I felt overwhelmed by the thought of a lifetime of medications, doctor's appointments, and restrictions.

But I refused to let this diagnosis define me. I embarked on a mission to take control of my health naturally, to lower my risk, reverse prediabetes, and protect my overall well-being. And now, I want to share everything I've learned with you.

In this comprehensive guide, I will walk you through a step-by-step program that will empower you to make positive changes in your life. Together, we will explore the power of natural prevention strategies that can transform your health and reduce your risk of developing Type 2 Diabetes.

Why focus on natural prevention, you may ask? Well, the truth is, our bodies are incredibly resilient and have an innate ability to heal themselves. By making simple yet effective lifestyle modifications, incorporating natural remedies, and adopting a holistic approach, you can take charge of your health and reclaim your vitality.

This book is not just about managing diabetes; it's about preventing it from ever taking hold. It's about equipping you with the knowledge, tools, and support you need to make informed decisions and create lasting change in your life.

Throughout the chapters, we will delve into various topics, such as assessing your risk, understanding prediabetes, implementing lifestyle modifications, exploring natural remedies and supplements, and creating a personalized prevention plan. We will also address frequently asked questions and provide you with practical tips to navigate this journey with confidence.

But remember, this is not a one-size-fits-all approach. We are all unique individuals with different needs and circumstances. That's why I encourage you to adapt the information in this book to suit your specific situation. Listen to your body, consult with healthcare professionals, and make choices that resonate with you.

I know that embarking on a journey towards optimal health can feel daunting, but I assure you, it is worth it. By taking small steps each day, you can transform your life and protect your health for years to come.

So, are you ready to join me on this empowering journey? Let's take the first step together and discover the incredible potential within you to prevent Type 2 Diabetes naturally.

Understanding Type 2 Diabetes

Type 2 diabetes is a chronic condition that affects the way your body metabolizes sugar (glucose), which is the main source of fuel for your cells. Unlike type 1 diabetes, which is an autoimmune disease that occurs when the body's immune system mistakenly attacks and destroys the insulin-producing cells in the pancreas, type 2 diabetes is primarily a result of lifestyle factors and genetic predisposition.

In type 2 diabetes, your body either doesn't produce enough insulin or becomes resistant to the insulin it does produce. Insulin is a hormone that helps regulate blood sugar levels by allowing glucose to enter your cells, where it can be used for energy. When insulin resistance occurs, glucose builds up in the bloodstream instead of being absorbed by the cells, leading to high blood sugar levels.

There are several factors that contribute to the development of type 2 diabetes, including:

1. Obesity: Excess body weight, especially around the abdomen, increases the risk of insulin resistance.

2. Physical Inactivity: Lack of regular physical activity can contribute to weight gain and insulin resistance.

3. Unhealthy Diet: Consuming a diet high in processed foods, sugary beverages, and saturated fats increases the risk of

developing type 2 diabetes.

4. Family History: Having a close family member, such as a parent or sibling, with type 2 diabetes increases your risk.

5. Age: The risk of developing type 2 diabetes increases with age, especially after the age of 45.

6. Ethnicity: Certain ethnic groups, such as African Americans, Hispanic/Latino Americans, Native Americans, and Asian Americans, have a higher risk of developing type 2 diabetes.

7. Gestational Diabetes: Women who have had gestational diabetes during pregnancy are at a higher risk of developing type 2 diabetes later in life.

Assessing Your Risk

Understanding your vulnerability to this chronic condition is the first step towards prevention and taking control of your health.

As someone who has personally experienced the impact of type 2 diabetes, I know how crucial it is to assess your risk factors. It was through this assessment that I gained valuable insights into my own susceptibility and was able to make informed decisions to protect my well-being.

So, let's dive in and explore the various risk factors for type 2 diabetes, including family history and genetics, lifestyle factors, and how you can assess your personal risk.

Risk Factors for Type 2 Diabetes:
Type 2 diabetes is a complex condition influenced by a combination of genetic, lifestyle, and environmental factors. By understanding these risk factors, we can gain a clearer picture of our susceptibility and take proactive measures to reduce our risk.

Family History and Genetics:

One significant risk factor for type 2 diabetes is a family history of the condition. If you have a parent, sibling, or close relative with type 2 diabetes, your risk increases. This suggests a genetic predisposition to the condition, although lifestyle factors also play a role.

While we cannot change our genetic makeup, being aware of our family history empowers us to take preventive measures. It serves as a reminder to be vigilant about our lifestyle choices and seek regular medical check-ups to catch any warning signs early.

Lifestyle Factors:
Lifestyle factors play a pivotal role in the development of type 2 diabetes. Certain habits and behaviors can significantly increase our risk, but the good news is that we have the power to make positive changes.

1. Unhealthy Diet: Consuming a diet high in processed foods, sugary beverages, saturated fats, and low in fiber can contribute to weight gain, insulin resistance, and ultimately, type 2 diabetes. Poor dietary choices can lead to obesity, a significant risk factor for the condition.

2. Physical Inactivity: Sedentary lifestyles devoid of regular physical activity can increase the risk of developing type 2 diabetes. Exercise helps maintain a healthy weight, improves insulin sensitivity, and promotes overall well-being.

3. Excess Weight and Obesity: Carrying excess weight, especially around the abdomen, is strongly associated with an

increased risk of type 2 diabetes. Fat cells release chemicals that can interfere with insulin's action, leading to insulin resistance.

4. High Blood Pressure and Cholesterol: Hypertension (high blood pressure) and high cholesterol levels are often seen in individuals with type 2 diabetes. These conditions can contribute to cardiovascular complications and further worsen diabetes management.

5. Smoking and Alcohol Consumption: Smoking and excessive alcohol consumption have been linked to an increased risk of type 2 diabetes. These habits can impair insulin sensitivity and damage blood vessels, exacerbating the condition.

Assessing Your Personal Risk:
Now that we have explored the various risk factors, it's time to assess your personal risk of developing type 2 diabetes. Remember, knowledge is power, and understanding your vulnerability allows you to take proactive steps towards prevention.

Here are some steps you can take to assess your risk:

1. Family History: Take note of your family history of type 2 diabetes. Talk to your parents, siblings, and close relatives to gather information about any instances of the condition. This will help you understand your genetic predisposition.

2. Health Check-ups: Schedule regular check-ups with your healthcare provider. They can evaluate your overall health, measure your blood sugar levels, and assess other risk factors such as blood pressure and cholesterol levels.

3. Body Mass Index (BMI): Calculate your BMI, which is a measure of body fat based on your height and weight. A BMI of 25 or higher indicates an increased risk of type 2 diabetes. However, keep in mind that BMI is not the sole determinant of risk, and other factors should be considered.

4. Waist Circumference: Measure your waist circumference using a tape measure. Excess abdominal fat is strongly associated with an increased risk of type 2 diabetes. For men, a waist circumference of 40 inches or more, and for women, 35 inches or more, indicates an elevated risk.

5. Symptoms and Warning Signs: Pay attention to any symptoms or warning signs that may indicate prediabetes or early-stage type 2 diabetes. These may include increased thirst, frequent urination, unexplained weight loss or gain, fatigue, blurred vision, or slow wound healing. If you experience any of these, consult your healthcare provider.

By assessing your personal risk, you can gain valuable insights into yourvulnerability to type 2 diabetes. This knowledge empowers you to make informed decisions and take proactive steps towards prevention.

Understanding Prediabetes

Prediabetes is a condition where blood sugar levels are higher than normal but not yet high enough to be diagnosed as type 2 diabetes. It's a critical warning sign that your body's metabolism is not functioning optimally and could lead to the development of type 2 diabetes if left untreated.

What is Prediabetes?

Prediabetes occurs when the body either doesn't produce enough insulin or becomes resistant to insulin's effects, resulting in elevated blood sugar levels. Insulin is a hormone produced by the pancreas that helps regulate blood sugar levels by allowing glucose to enter cells for energy. When this process is impaired, glucose accumulates in the bloodstream, leading to prediabetes.

Signs and Symptoms

Prediabetes often doesn't present any noticeable symptoms, which is why it's crucial to undergo regular screenings, especially if you have risk factors such as being overweight, having a sedentary lifestyle, or a family history of diabetes. However, some individuals may experience symptoms such as increased thirst, frequent urination, fatigue, and blurred vision.

Diagnosis and Testing

Prediabetes is typically diagnosed through blood tests that measure fasting blood sugar levels or HbA1c levels. A fasting blood sugar level between 100 and 125 mg/dL (5.6 to 6.9 mmol/L) indicates prediabetes, while an HbA1c level between 5.7% and 6.4% is also indicative of prediabetes. These tests are essential for early detection and intervention to prevent the progression to type 2 diabetes.

The Link Between Prediabetes and Type 2 Diabetes

Prediabetes is a significant risk factor for developing type 2 diabetes. Without intervention, up to 70% of individuals with prediabetes may progress to type 2 diabetes within a decade. Additionally, prediabetes is associated with an increased risk of cardiovascular disease, stroke, and other complications.

Several factors contribute to the development of prediabetes, including genetics, obesity, physical inactivity, and poor diet. Fortunately, lifestyle modifications such as adopting a healthy diet, increasing physical activity, and maintaining a healthy weight can significantly reduce the risk of developing type 2 diabetes.

Prediabetes serves as a crucial warning sign for individuals to take proactive steps towards improving their health and preventing the onset of type 2 diabetes. By understanding the risk factors, recognizing the signs and symptoms, and undergoing regular screenings, individuals can make informed decisions to manage their blood sugar levels and lead healthier lives. Early intervention through lifestyle changes and, in some cases, medication, can help reverse prediabetes and reduce the risk of developing type 2 diabetes and its complications.

Lifestyle Modifications for Prevention

By making simple yet effective changes to our daily routines, we can significantly reduce our risk of developing type 2 diabetes and improve our overall health and well-being.

Healthy Eating Habits

One of the cornerstones of diabetes prevention is adopting healthy eating habits. A balanced and nutritious diet plays a vital role in maintaining stable blood sugar levels and promoting optimal health. Here are some key principles to keep in mind:

1. Choose whole, unprocessed foods: Opt for fresh fruits, vegetables, whole grains, lean proteins, and healthy fats. These foods are rich in essential nutrients and fiber, which can help regulate blood sugar levels and promote satiety.

2. Limit refined sugars and carbohydrates: Minimize your intake of sugary beverages, candies, pastries, and processed foods that are high in refined sugars and carbohydrates. These can cause rapid spikes in blood sugar levels and contribute to insulin resistance.

3. Focus on portion control: Be mindful of your portion sizes and aim for balanced meals that include a variety of food groups. This can help prevent overeating and promote better blood sugar control.

4. Monitor carbohydrate intake: Pay attention to the types and amounts of carbohydrates you consume. Complex carbohydrates, such as whole grains, legumes, and vegetables, are preferable over simple carbohydrates, like white bread and sugary snacks.

5. Stay hydrated: Drink plenty of water throughout the day to stay hydrated and support overall health. Limit your consumption of sugary beverages, as they can contribute to weight gain and increase the risk of diabetes.

Healthy eating is not about strict diets or deprivation. It's about nourishing your body with wholesome foods that provide the nutrients it needs to function optimally.

The Role of Physical Activity

Regular physical activity is another crucial component of diabetes prevention. Exercise helps improve insulin sensitivity, promotes weight loss or maintenance, and enhances overall cardiovascular health. Here are some tips to incorporate physical activity into your daily routine:

1. Find activities you enjoy: Choose activities that you genuinely enjoy, whether it's walking, cycling, dancing, swimming, or playing a sport. This will make it easier to stay motivated

and consistent.

2. Set realistic goals: Start with small, achievable goals and gradually increase the intensity and duration of your workouts. Aim for at least 150 minutes of moderate-intensity aerobic activity per week, along with strength training exercises twice a week.

3. Make it a habit: Schedule regular exercise sessions into your weekly routine and treat them as non-negotiable appointments with yourself. Consistency is key to reaping the long-term benefits of physical activity.

4. Stay active throughout the day: Look for opportunities to incorporate movement into your daily life. Take the stairs instead of the elevator, go for short walks during breaks, or engage in active hobbies like gardening or dancing.

5. Listen to your body: Pay attention to how your body feels during and after exercise. If you experience any pain or discomfort, modify your activities or seek guidance from a healthcare professional.

Remember, physical activity doesn't have to be strenuous or complicated. Find what works for you and make it a priority to move your body regularly.

Stress Management Techniques

Chronic stress can have a detrimental impact on our health, including an increased risk of developing type 2 diabetes.

Therefore, incorporating stress management techniques into our daily lives is essential for prevention. Here are some effective strategies:

1. Practice relaxation techniques: Engage in activities that promote relaxation, such as deep breathing exercises, meditation, yoga, or tai chi. These practices can help reduce stress hormones and promote a sense of calm.

2. Prioritize self-care: Make time for activities that bring you joy and help you unwind. This could include hobbies, spending time in nature, reading, taking baths, or listening to music. Taking care of your mental and emotional well-being is crucial for overall health.

3. Establish healthy boundaries: Learn to say no when necessary and set boundaries to protect your time and energy. Overcommitting yourself can lead to increased stress levels and a neglect of self-care.

4. Seek support: Reach out to friends, family, or support groups for emotional support. Sometimes, talking about our stressors and concerns can provide relief and perspective.

5. Engage in regular exercise: Physical activity not only benefits our physical health but also acts as a powerful stress reliever. Incorporate exercise into your routine to help manage stress levels effectively.

Stress is a part of life, but how we respond to it can make a significant difference in our overall well-being. By implementing stress management techniques, we can reduce the impact of stress on our bodies and lower our risk of developing type 2 diabetes.

Importance of Quality Sleep

Sleep plays a vital role in maintaining overall health and well-being. Poor sleep quality or insufficientsleep duration can disrupt hormonal balance, increase insulin resistance, and contribute to weight gain, all of which are risk factors for type 2 diabetes. Here are some tips for improving sleep quality:

1. Establish a bedtime routine: Create a relaxing routine before bed to signal to your body that it's time to wind down. This could include activities such as reading, taking a warm bath, or practicing relaxation techniques.

2. Create a sleep-friendly environment: Make your bedroom a comfortable and peaceful space. Keep the room cool, dark, and quiet, and invest in a supportive mattress and pillows.

3. Limit exposure to screens: The blue light emitted by electronic devices can interfere with your sleep. Avoid using screens, such as smartphones, tablets, and laptops, for at least an hour before bed.

4. Stick to a consistent sleep schedule: Try to go to bed and wake up at the same time every day, even on weekends. This helps regulate your body's internal clock and promotes better sleep quality.

5. Avoid stimulants close to bedtime: Limit your consumption of caffeine and avoid heavy meals, nicotine, and alcohol close to bedtime, as they can disrupt sleep patterns.

6. Manage stress: As mentioned earlier, stress can interfere with sleep. Incorporate stress management techniques into your daily routine to promote better sleep quality.

7. Create a comfortable sleep environment: Invest in a supportive mattress and pillows, use blackout curtains or an eye mask to block out light, and use earplugs or a white noise machine to drown out any disruptive sounds.

By prioritizing quality sleep and implementing these strategies, you can improve your overall health and reduce your risk of developing type 2 diabetes.

Natural Remedies and Supplements

In this chapter, we will explore the power of natural remedies and supplements in supporting diabetes prevention. While lifestyle modifications are the foundation of prevention, certain herbs, nutrients, and supplements can provide additional support in managing blood sugar levels and promoting overall health. Join us as we delve into the world of natural remedies and discover their potential benefits in the fight against type 2 diabetes.

Herbal Remedies for Blood Sugar Control

In the quest for natural solutions to support blood sugar control, herbal remedies have gained significant attention. These plant-based remedies have been used for centuries in traditional medicine systems and are now being studied for their potential benefits in managing blood sugar levels. While it's important to consult with a healthcare professional before incorporating any new herbal remedies into your routine, here are a few herbs that have shown promise in supporting blood sugar control:

1. Cinnamon

Cinnamon is a popular spice known for its sweet and warm flavor. It has been used in traditional medicine to help regulate blood sugar levels. Studies have shown that cinnamon may improve insulin sensitivity and enhance the body's ability to use glucose effectively. It may also help reduce fasting blood sugar levels. Incorporating cinnamon into your diet can be as simple as sprinkling it on oatmeal, adding it to smoothies, or using it in baking.

2. Gymnema Sylvestre

Gymnema Sylvestre is an herb native to India and has been used in Ayurvedic medicine for its potential blood sugar-lowering effects. It is believed to work by reducing sugar cravings and inhibiting the absorption of sugar in the intestines. Gymnema Sylvestre may also support insulin production and improve glucose utilization. This herb is available in supplement form and should be taken under the guidance of a healthcare professional.

3. Fenugreek

Fenugreek is a spice commonly used in Indian cuisine and has been studied for its potential benefits in blood sugar control. It contains soluble fiber and compounds that may help slow down the digestion and absorption of carbohydrates, resulting in improved blood sugar levels. Fenugreek may also enhance insulin sensitivity and reduce insulin resistance. It can be consumed as a spice, brewed into tea, or taken in supplement form.

4. Ginseng

Ginseng is a popular herb in traditional Chinese medicine and has been studied for its potential effects on blood sugar control. Both American and Asian ginseng have shown promise in improving insulin sensitivity and reducing blood sugar levels. Ginseng may also have antioxidant properties that help protect against diabetes-related complications. It is available in various forms, including capsules, powders, and teas.

5. Aloe Vera

Aloe Vera is a succulent plant known for its gel-like substance that is commonly used for skin care. However, it may also have potential benefits in blood sugar control. Some studies suggest that Aloe Vera may help lower fasting blood sugar levels and improve insulin sensitivity. It is important to note that Aloe Vera should be used with caution, as it can interact with certain medications and may have laxative effects. Consult with a healthcare professional before using Aloe Vera for blood sugar control.

While these herbal remedies show promise in supporting blood sugar control, it's essential to remember that they are not a substitute for a healthy lifestyle and medical advice. It's important to work with a healthcare professional to determine the right dosage, potential interactions, and overall suitability of these herbs for your individual needs.

Vitamins and Minerals for Diabetes Prevention

In addition to herbal remedies, certain vitamins and minerals play a crucial role in supporting diabetes prevention. These essential nutrients are involved in various metabolic processes and can help regulate blood sugar levels. While a balanced diet should provide most of these nutrients, some individuals may benefit from supplementation. Let's explore the key vitamins and minerals that can support your diabetes prevention journey:

1. Vitamin D

Vitamin D is not only essential for bone health but also plays a role in blood sugar regulation. Research suggests that vitamin D deficiency may increase the risk of developing type 2 diabetes. Adequate vitamin D levels have been associated with improved insulin sensitivity and lower fasting blood sugar levels. While sunlight is the best source of vitamin D, supplementation may be necessary for individuals with limited sun exposure or those with low levels.

2. Magnesium

Magnesium is involved in over 300 biochemical reactions in the body, including carbohydrate metabolism and insulin action. Studies have shown that magnesium deficiency is associated with an increased risk of developing type 2 diabetes. Adequate magnesium intake may improve insulin sensitivity and help regulate blood sugar levels. Good dietary sources of magnesium include leafy green vegetables, nuts, seeds, and whole grains.

3. Chromium

Chromium is a mineral that plays a role in insulin action and glucose metabolism. It helps enhance the effectiveness of insulin in transporting glucose into cells. Some studies suggest that chromium supplementation may improve blood sugar control and insulin sensitivity in individuals with type 2 diabetes. Good dietary sources of chromium include broccoli, whole grains, and lean meats.

4. B Vitamins

B vitamins, including B1 (thiamine), B6 (pyridoxine), and B12 (cobalamin), are essential for energy metabolism and nerve function. They also play a role in blood sugar regulation. Thiamine deficiency, in particular, has been associated with an increased risk of developing diabetes. B vitamin supplementation may help improve glucose metabolism and reduce the risk of diabetic complications. Good dietary sources of B vitamins include whole grains, legumes, leafy greens, and animal products.

5. Zinc

Zinc is involved in insulin synthesis, storage, and secretion. It also plays a role in the metabolism of carbohydrates, proteins, and fats. Studies have shown that zinc deficiency may impair insulin function and increase the risk of developing diabetes. Adequate zinc intake may help improve insulin sensitivity and support healthy blood sugar control. Good dietary sources of zinc include oysters, beef, poultry, nuts, and seeds.

It's important to note that while these vitamins and minerals can support blood sugar control, they should not replace a balanced diet or medical advice. It's always best to obtain nutrients from whole foods whenever possible. If you're considering supplementation, consult with a healthcare professional to determine the appropriate dosage and ensure it aligns with your individual needs.

Omega-3 Fatty Acids and Diabetes

Omega-3 fatty acids are a type of polyunsaturated fat that is renowned for its numerous health benefits. These essential fats are found in fatty fish, such as salmon, mackerel, and sardines, as well as in certain plant-based sources like flaxseeds and walnuts. In recent years, research has explored the potential role of omega-3 fatty acids in diabetes prevention and management. Let's delve into the relationship between omega-3 fatty acids and diabetes:

1. Improved Insulin Sensitivity

Insulin sensitivity refers to the body's ability to respond to insulin and effectively regulate blood sugar levels. Studies have suggested that omega-3 fatty acids may improve insulin sensitivity, which is beneficial for individuals with type 2 diabetes or those at risk of developing the condition. By enhancing insulin sensitivity, omega-3 fatty acids may help improve glucose uptake by cells, leading to better blood sugar control.

2. Reduced Inflammation

Chronic inflammation is believed to play a significant role in the development of insulin resistance and type 2 diabetes. Omega-3 fatty acids possess anti-inflammatory properties that can help reduce inflammation in the body. By decreasing inflammation, omega-3 fatty acids may contribute to improved insulin sensitivity and reduced risk of diabetes.

3. Cardiovascular Health Benefits

Individuals with diabetes are at a higher risk of developing cardiovascular complications. Omega-3 fatty acids have been shown to have positive effects on heart health by reducing triglyceride levels, lowering blood pressure, and improving overall cardiovascular function. By supporting cardiovascular health, omega-3 fatty acids may help mitigate the risk of diabetes-related heart complications.

4. Potential Weight Management Aid

Maintaining a healthy weight is crucial for diabetes prevention and management. Omega-3 fatty acids may play a role in weight management by promoting satiety, reducing appetite, and increasing fat oxidation. By incorporating omega-3-rich foods into your diet, you may feel more satisfied after meals, which can help prevent overeating and support weight control.

5. Eye Health

Diabetes can have detrimental effects on eye health, leading to conditions such as diabetic retinopathy. Omega-3 fatty acids have been associated with a reduced risk of developing certain eye diseases. These healthy fats may help protect the retina and maintain optimal eye health, which is particularly important for individuals with diabetes.

While omega-3 fatty acids show promise in diabetes prevention and management, it's important to note that they should not replace other essential aspects of diabetes care, such as medication, a balanced diet, regular exercise, and medical supervision. Incorporating omega-3-rich foods into your diet, such as fatty fish, flaxseeds, chia seeds, and walnuts, can be a beneficial addition to your overall diabetes prevention strategy.

In the next section, we will address some frequently asked questions related to natural remedies, supplements, and lifestyle modifications for diabetes prevention. Stay tuned for expert answers to common queries.

Probiotics and Gut Health

Probiotics are live microorganisms that provide health benefits when consumed in adequate amounts. These beneficial bacteria are commonly found in fermented foods like yogurt, sauerkraut, and kimchi, as well as in supplement form. While probiotics are often associated with digestive health, their impact extends beyond the gut. Let's explore the relationship between probiotics and gut health:

1. Restoring and Maintaining Gut Microbiota Balance

The gut microbiota is a complex community of microorganisms that reside in the digestive tract. A healthy gut microbiota is essential for proper digestion, nutrient absorption, immune function, and overall well-being. However, factors such as poor diet, stress, antibiotics, and illness can disrupt the balance of gut bacteria. Probiotics can help restore and maintain a healthy gut microbiota by introducing beneficial bacteria into the digestive system.

2. Improved Digestive Function

Probiotics play a crucial role in promoting healthy digestion. They help break down food, enhance nutrient absorption, and support the production of enzymes that aid in digestion. Probiotics can also help alleviate symptoms of digestive disorders such as irritable bowel syndrome (IBS), inflammatory bowel disease (IBD), and diarrhea. By improving digestive function, probiotics contribute to overall gut health.

3. Enhanced Immune Function

A significant portion of the immune system resides in the gut. Probiotics can stimulate the production of immune cells and enhance their activity, thereby strengthening the immune response. By supporting immune function, probiotics may help reduce the risk of infections and promote overall health and well-being.

4. Reduced Inflammation

Chronic inflammation in the gut can contribute to various

digestive disorders and even systemic health issues. Probiotics have been shown to have anti-inflammatory properties, helping to reduce inflammation in the gut. By reducing gut inflammation, probiotics may alleviate symptoms of conditions such as Crohn's disease, ulcerative colitis, and other inflammatory bowel diseases.

5. Mental Health and Brain Function

Emerging research suggests a strong connection between the gut and the brain, known as the gut-brain axis. Probiotics can influence the gut-brain axis by producing neurotransmitters and other bioactive compounds that affect brain function and mood. Some studies have shown that probiotics may help improve symptoms of anxiety, depression, and stress-related disorders. By supporting a healthy gut, probiotics may positively impact mental health.

It's important to note that not all probiotics are the same, and their effectiveness can vary depending on the strain and dosage. When choosing a probiotic supplement, look for products that contain specific strains with proven benefits for the condition you are targeting. It's also advisable to consult with a healthcare professional to determine the most suitable probiotic for your individual needs.

Incorporating probiotic-rich foods into your diet, such as yogurt, kefir, tempeh, and kombucha, can also be a beneficial way to support gut health. Remember to opt for products that contain live and active cultures to ensure the presence of beneficial bacteria.

Creating a Personalized Prevention Plan

This plan should be tailored to your individual needs, taking into account your lifestyle, preferences, and goals. In this chapter, we will explore important aspects of creating a personalized prevention plan, including setting realistic goals, tracking progress, seeking professional guidance, and building a support system.

Setting Realistic Goals

Setting realistic goals is crucial when it comes to diabetes prevention. It's important to establish achievable objectives that align with your current health status and lifestyle. Setting unrealistic goals can lead to frustration and a higher likelihood of giving up. Start by identifying specific behaviors or habits that you want to change, such as improving your diet, increasing physical activity, or managing stress levels. Break these goals down into smaller, actionable steps that can be easily integrated into your daily routine. By setting realistic goals, you can maintain motivation and track your progress effectively.

Tracking Progress

Tracking your progress is an essential part of any prevention plan. It allows you to monitor your efforts, identify areas of improvement, and celebrate your successes. There are various ways to track your progress, depending on your preferences and the goals you've set. You can use a journal or a mobile app to record your daily food intake, physical activity, and other relevant data. Regularly measuring and recording your weight, blood pressure, and blood sugar levels can also provide valuable insights into your progress. By tracking your progress, you can stay accountable and make necessary adjustments to your prevention plan.

Seeking Professional Guidance

Seeking professional guidance is highly recommended when creating a personalized prevention plan. Healthcare professionals, such as doctors, dietitians, and fitness trainers, can provide expert advice and support. They can help you assess your current health status, identify potential risk factors, and develop a tailored prevention plan. These professionals can also guide you in making informed decisions regarding diet, exercise, medication (if necessary), and lifestyle modifications. By seeking professional guidance, you can ensure that your prevention plan is based on accurate information and tailored to your specific needs.

Building a Support System

Building a support system is essential for long-term success in diabetes prevention. Surrounding yourself with supportive individuals who understand and encourage your goals can make a significant difference in your journey. Share your prevention plan with family, friends, and colleagues, and explain why it's important to you. Seek their support and understanding, as they can help create a positive environment that fosters healthy habits. Consider joining support groups or online communities focused on diabetes prevention. These platforms provide opportunities to connect with others who are on a similar path, share experiences, and exchange valuable tips. By building a support system, you can stay motivated, accountable, and inspired throughout your prevention journey.

Remember, creating a personalized prevention plan is a dynamic process. It may require adjustments along the way as you learn more about your body, preferences, and what works best for you. Be open to adapting your plan as needed and stay committed to your goals. With realistic goals, consistent progress tracking, professional guidance, and a strong support system, you can take control of your health and effectively prevent diabetes.

Long-Term Strategies for Diabetes Prevention

In the pursuit of diabetes prevention, it's essential to adopt long-term strategies that promote overall health and well-being. These strategies include maintaining a healthy weight, regular monitoring of blood sugar levels, managing stress and emotional well-being, and staying committed to a healthy lifestyle.

Maintaining a Healthy Weight

Maintaining a healthy weight is crucial for diabetes prevention. Excess weight, especially around the waistline, increases the risk of developing type 2 diabetes. By achieving and maintaining a healthy weight, you can improve insulin sensitivity and reduce the strain on your body's ability to regulate blood sugar levels. Incorporate a balanced diet rich in fruits, vegetables, whole grains, lean proteins, and healthy fats. Avoid sugary beverages, processed foods, and excessive calorie intake. Regular physical activity is also essential for weight management. Aim for at least 150 minutes of moderate-intensity exercise per week, such as brisk walking, cycling, or swimming.

Regular Monitoring of Blood Sugar Levels

Regular monitoring of blood sugar levels is vital for diabetes prevention. It allows you to stay informed about your body's glucose levels and detect any potential abnormalities early on. If you have prediabetes or are at risk of developing diabetes, your healthcare provider may recommend periodic blood sugar tests. These tests can help assess your risk level and guide you in making necessary lifestyle modifications. By monitoring your blood sugar levels, you can take proactive steps to prevent the progression of prediabetes to type 2 diabetes.

Managing Stress and Emotional Well-being

Stress and emotional well-being play a significant role in diabetes prevention. Chronic stress can contribute to unhealthy behaviors, such as overeating, poor food choices, and sedentary lifestyle habits, which increase the risk of developing diabetes. Find healthy ways to manage stress, such as practicing relaxation techniques, engaging in regular physical activity, getting enough sleep, and seeking support from loved ones. Prioritize self-care activities that promote emotional well-being, such as hobbies, mindfulness practices, and spending time in nature. By managing stress and prioritizing emotional well-being, you can reduce the risk of diabetes and improve overall health.

Staying Committed to a Healthy Lifestyle

Staying committed to a healthy lifestyle is essential for long-term diabetes prevention. It's not just about making temporary changes but adopting sustainable habits that become part of your daily routine. Make healthy choices a priority in your life by consistently following a balanced diet, engaging in regular physical activity, and practicing self-care. Surround yourself with a supportive environment that encourages healthy behaviors and holds you accountable. Celebrate your successes along the way and stay motivated by setting new goals and challenging yourself. By staying committed to a healthy lifestyle, you can significantly reduce the risk of developing diabetes and enjoy a higher quality of life.

Frequently Asked Questions (FAQ)

<u>Question 1: Can Type 2 Diabetes be Prevented?</u>

Absolutely! Type 2 diabetes can be prevented or delayed through various lifestyle modifications and healthy habits. Research has shown that making positive changes in diet, physical activity, and overall lifestyle can significantly reduce the risk of developing type 2 diabetes, especially for individuals with prediabetes.

By adopting a healthy eating plan that focuses on whole foods, including fruits, vegetables, whole grains, lean proteins, and healthy fats, you can improve your insulin sensitivity and maintain stable blood sugar levels. Avoiding sugary beverages, processed foods, and excessive calorie intake is also crucial.

Regular physical activity is another key component in diabetes prevention. Engaging in moderate-intensity exercise for at least 150 minutes per week can help control weight, improve insulin sensitivity, and lower the risk of developing diabetes. Find activities that you enjoy and make them a regular part of your routine.

Additionally, maintaining a healthy weight is essential for

diabetes prevention. Losing excess weight, especially around the waistline, can significantly reduce the risk of developing type 2 diabetes. Combining a balanced diet with regular physical activity is the most effective approach to achieving and maintaining a healthy weight.

It's important to note that while lifestyle modifications can greatly reduce the risk of type 2 diabetes, there are other factors such as genetics and family history that may also contribute to the development of the disease. However, by making positive changes and adopting a proactive approach to your health, you can significantly lower your risk and potentially prevent type 2 diabetes altogether.

Question 2: What are the Early Warning Signs of Diabetes?

Recognizing the early warning signs of diabetes is crucial for early detection and intervention. While the symptoms may vary from person to person, there are common signs that can indicate the presence of diabetes. It's important to note that these symptoms may also be associated with other health conditions, so it's essential to consult with a healthcare professional for an accurate diagnosis. Here are some early warning signs of diabetes:

1. Frequent urination: If you find yourself urinating more frequently than usual, especially waking up multiple times during the night to urinate, it could be a sign of diabetes. Excess glucose in the blood can cause the kidneys to work harder to filter and remove the sugar, leading to increased urination.

2. Excessive thirst: Feeling constantly thirsty, even after

drinking an adequate amount of fluids, can be a sign of diabetes. The increased urination caused by high blood sugar levels can lead to dehydration, triggering the feeling of excessive thirst.

3. Unexplained weight loss: Sudden and unexplained weight loss, despite normal or increased appetite, can be a warning sign of diabetes. When the body doesn't have enough insulin or is unable to use it properly, it may start breaking down muscle and fat for energy, resulting in weight loss.

4. Fatigue and weakness: Feeling excessively tired, fatigued, or lacking energy, even after getting enough rest, can be a symptom of diabetes. High blood sugar levels can affect the body's ability to convert glucose into energy, leading to feelings of fatigue and weakness.

5. Blurred vision: Diabetes can affect the eyes and cause changes in vision. Blurred vision, difficulty focusing, or experiencing sudden changes in eyesight may be early warning signs of diabetes. High blood sugar levels can cause fluid imbalances in the eyes, affecting their ability to focus properly.

Question 3: Are There Any Natural Remedies for Diabetes Prevention?

While there are no natural remedies that can guarantee the prevention of diabetes, certain lifestyle practices and natural approaches can help reduce the risk and support overall health. It's important to note that these methods should not replace medical advice or prescribed treatments. Here are some natural approaches that may aid in diabetes prevention:

1. Healthy Diet: Adopting a healthy and balanced diet is key to diabetes prevention. Focus on consuming whole foods, including fruits, vegetables, whole grains, lean proteins, and healthy fats. Avoid processed foods, sugary snacks, and beverages. Incorporate foods with low glycemic index (GI) that have a minimal impact on blood sugar levels.

2. Regular Physical Activity: Engaging in regular exercise is beneficial for diabetes prevention. Aim for at least 150 minutes of moderate-intensity aerobic activity per week, such as brisk walking, cycling, or swimming. Physical activity helps improve insulin sensitivity, manage weight, and maintain overall health.

3. Stress Management: Chronic stress can contribute to the development of diabetes. Practice stress management techniques such as meditation, deep breathing exercises, yoga, or engaging in hobbies that help you relax. Prioritizing self-care and finding healthy outlets for stress can support overall well-being.

4. Herbal Supplements: Some herbal supplements may have potential benefits for diabetes prevention, but it's important to consult with a healthcare professional before taking any supplements. Examples include cinnamon, fenugreek, bitter melon, and aloe vera. These herbs have been studied for their potential effects on blood sugar control, but more research is needed to establish their efficacy.

5. Maintain a Healthy Weight: Maintaining a healthy weight is crucial for diabetes prevention. Focus on achieving and maintaining a weight that is appropriate for your body type and

height. A combination of a healthy diet and regular physical activity can help in weight management.

<u>Question 4: How Can I Lower My Risk of Developing Prediabetes?</u>

Lowering your risk of developing prediabetes involves making positive lifestyle changes and adopting healthy habits. Prediabetes is a condition where blood sugar levels are higher than normal but not yet in the range of diabetes. By taking proactive steps, you can prevent or delay the progression to type 2 diabetes. Here are some strategies to lower your risk of developing prediabetes:

1. Maintain a Healthy Weight: Losing excess weight and maintaining a healthy weight is one of the most effective ways to lower your risk of prediabetes. Focus on achieving a body mass index (BMI) within the healthy range for your height and body type. Even a modest weight loss of 5-10% can have significant benefits.

2. Eat a Balanced Diet: Adopting a balanced and nutritious diet is crucial for lowering the risk of prediabetes. Include a variety of fruits, vegetables, whole grains, lean proteins, and healthy fats in your meals. Limit your intake of sugary foods, processed snacks, and beverages high in added sugars.

3. Engage in Regular Physical Activity: Regular exercise is essential for lowering the risk of prediabetes. Aim for at least 150 minutes of moderate-intensity aerobic activity per week, such as brisk walking, jogging, cycling, or swimming. Additionally, incorporate strength training exercises to build

muscle and improve overall fitness.

4. Limit Sedentary Behavior: Reduce the amount of time spent sitting or being sedentary. Prolonged sitting has been linked to an increased risk of prediabetes and type 2 diabetes. Take frequent breaks from sitting, stand up and stretch, and incorporate movement throughout your day.

5. Manage Stress: Chronic stress can contribute to the development of prediabetes. Find healthy ways to manage stress, such as practicing relaxation techniques, engaging in hobbies, or seeking support from loved ones. Prioritize self-care and make time for activities that bring you joy and relaxation.

6. Get Regular Check-ups: Regular check-ups with your healthcare provider are essential for monitoring your health and detecting any signs of prediabetes. They can perform blood tests to assess your blood sugar levels and provide guidance on managing your risk factors.

Question 5: Is Type 2 Diabetes Reversible?

Yes, type 2 diabetes can be reversible in some cases. While it is a chronic condition, meaning it lasts a lifetime, with proper management and lifestyle changes, it is possible to achieve normal blood sugar levels and reduce or eliminate the need for medication.

The key to reversing type 2 diabetes lies in adopting a healthy lifestyle that focuses on diet, exercise, and weight management. Here are some strategies that can help in reversing type 2 diabetes:

1. Healthy Eating: Following a balanced and nutritious diet is crucial for managing and potentially reversing type 2 diabetes. Focus on consuming whole foods, including fruits, vegetables, whole grains, lean proteins, and healthy fats. Limit your intake of processed foods, sugary snacks, and beverages high in added sugars. Consider working with a registered dietitian to create a personalized meal plan.

2. Regular Physical Activity: Engaging in regular exercise is essential for managing blood sugar levels and improving insulin sensitivity. Aim for at least 150 minutes of moderate-intensity aerobic activity per week, such as brisk walking, jogging, cycling, or swimming. Additionally, incorporate strength training exercises to build muscle and improve overall fitness.

3. Weight Management: Losing excess weight, especially around the waistline, can have a significant impact on reversing type 2 diabetes. Excess weight contributes to insulin resistance, making it harder for the body to regulate blood sugar levels. By achieving and maintaining a healthy weight, you can improve insulin sensitivity and better manage diabetes.

4. Medication and Insulin: In some cases, medication or insulin may be necessary to manage blood sugar levels. However, as you make lifestyle changes and improve your overall health, it is possible to reduce or eliminate the need for medication under the guidance of your healthcare provider. It's important to work closely with your healthcare team to determine the

best approach for your specific situation.

It's important to note that the ability to reverse type 2 diabetes may vary from person to person. Factors such as the duration of the condition, individual response to lifestyle changes, and overall health play a role. Reversal is more likely in the early stages of the disease and for individuals who are proactive in adopting a healthy lifestyle.

Conclusion

"Type 2 Diabetes Natural Prevention Guide" serves as a comprehensive resource for individuals looking to take control of their health and prevent the onset of type 2 diabetes. Throughout this book, we have explored various natural approaches, lifestyle changes, and strategies that can significantly reduce the risk of developing this chronic condition.

By emphasizing the importance of a healthy diet, regular physical activity, stress management, and weight control, this guide empowers readers to make positive changes in their lives. It encourages them to embrace a holistic approach to their well-being, recognizing that prevention is not only possible but within their reach.

Taking control of one's health requires dedication, commitment, and a willingness to make sustainable lifestyle changes. This book aims to provide the necessary knowledge, tools, and encouragement to embark on this journey. It emphasizes the power of small steps and gradual progress, reminding readers that every positive choice they make contributes to their overall health and well-being.

By adopting the principles outlined in this guide, individuals can not only reduce their risk of developing type 2 diabetes but also improve their overall quality of life. It is a reminder that our health is in our hands, and with the right information and support, we can make a significant impact on our well-being.

In closing, "Type 2 Diabetes Natural Prevention Guide" serves as a beacon of hope and encouragement for individuals seeking to take control of their health. It reminds us that prevention is possible, and by making conscious choices, we can pave the way for a healthier, happier future. Let this guide be your companion on your journey towards optimal health and well-being.

Remember, you have the power to make a difference in your life. Take the first step today and embrace the path to natural prevention of type 2 diabetes.

Thanks

Thank you, dear reader, for taking the time to delve into the pages of "Type 2 Diabetes Natural Prevention Guide." I hope that the information and insights shared within these chapters have been valuable to you on your journey towards better health.

If you found this book helpful and informative, I kindly ask you to consider leaving a review and sharing your thoughts. Your feedback will not only help me improve as a writer but also assist others in deciding whether this guide is right for them. Your support is greatly appreciated.

Furthermore, I encourage you to share this book with your loved ones, friends, and anyone who may benefit from the knowledge and strategies presented here. By spreading the word, you can contribute to a healthier and more informed community.

Remember, taking control of your health is a continuous process, and it is my sincere hope that "Type 2 Diabetes Natural Prevention Guide" has provided you with the encouragement and tools to make positive changes in your life. Together, let us strive for a future where diabetes prevention becomes a reality for all.

Thank you once again for your readership and support.